Table of content

A. Exploring the science of sleep and its benefits

B. The impact of stress and anxiety on sleep quality

C. Uncovering the connection between relaxation and overall well-being

III. The Fundamentals of Meditation and Mindfulness

A. Defining meditation and mindfulness

B. Brief history and cultural context of these practices

C. How meditation and mindfulness contribute

to better sleep and relaxation

IV. Preparing for Better Sleep and Relaxation

A. Creating a conducive sleep environment

B. Establishing a consistent bedtime routine

C. Addressing common obstacles to quality sleep and relaxation

V. Techniques for Mindful Sleep

A. Mindfulness of the breath and body

B. Progressive muscle relaxation for deep rest

C. Guided imagery
and visualization for
peaceful sleep

VI. Meditation
Practices for Relaxation

A. Mindful awareness
of thoughts and
emotions

B. Loving-kindness
meditation for self-
compassion and stress
reduction

C. Body scan
meditation for
releasing tension and
promoting relaxation

VII. Integrating
Meditation and
Mindfulness into Daily
Life

A. Applying mindfulness to daily activities for increased relaxation

B. Cultivating gratitude and joy through mindfulness

C. Managing stress and anxiety through regular meditation practice

VIII. Overcoming Challenges and Sustaining Practice

A. Dealing with restlessness and wandering thoughts during meditation

B. Strategies for maintaining motivation and consistency

A. How diet and nutrition influence sleep quality

B. Exercise and its impact on sleep and relaxation

C. Mindfulness-based stress reduction techniques for better sleep

XI. Enhancing Sleep and Relaxation for Specific Populations

A. Meditative practices for children and adolescents

B. Meditation and mindfulness for older adults

C. Addressing sleep disorders through

meditation and
mindfulness

XII. Conclusion

A. Recap of key
concepts and
techniques covered in
the book

B. Encouragement for
readers to embark on
their own meditation
and mindfulness
journey

C. Final thoughts on
the transformative
power of sleep and
relaxation through
meditation

Introduction:

In today's fast-paced world, where the demands of work, technology, and daily responsibilities can be overwhelming, finding a sense of calm and tranquility is essential for our well-being. Sleep and relaxation play a crucial role in maintaining our physical health, mental clarity, and emotional balance. However, achieving deep, restorative sleep and genuine relaxation can sometimes feel like an elusive dream.

Fortunately, there is a powerful tool that can help us reclaim our nights of peaceful slumber and create a sanctuary of relaxation in our lives: meditation and mindfulness. These ancient practices have been celebrated for their ability to quiet the mind, reduce stress, and promote a profound sense of calm. By integrating meditation and mindfulness into our daily routines, we can unlock the gateway to better sleep and enhanced relaxation.

This eBook, "Meditation and Mindfulness Practices for Better Sleep and Relaxation," is a comprehensive guide that explores the transformative potential of these practices. It delves into the science behind sleep, the impact of stress on our rest, and the undeniable connection between relaxation and overall well-being. Drawing upon the wisdom of meditation and mindfulness, it offers practical techniques and strategies to help you cultivate a

peaceful mind and a
restful body.

Throughout this book,
we will navigate the
fundamentals of
meditation and
mindfulness, providing
a clear understanding
of these practices and
their historical context.
We will explore how
meditation and
mindfulness contribute
to better sleep and
relaxation, unraveling
the profound ways in
which they influence
our mental and
physical states.

To facilitate your
journey towards

improved sleep and relaxation, we will guide you through the process of creating an optimal sleep environment, establishing a consistent bedtime routine, and addressing common obstacles that hinder quality rest. We will also introduce techniques specifically designed to promote mindful sleep, such as breath awareness, progressive muscle relaxation, and guided imagery.

Moreover, we will delve into meditation practices tailored for relaxation, offering guidance on cultivating mindful awareness of thoughts and emotions, practicing loving-kindness meditation for self-compassion, and releasing tension through body scan meditation. These techniques will empower you to integrate mindfulness into your daily life, discovering how it can enhance various activities, cultivate gratitude and joy, and effectively manage stress and anxiety.

We understand that maintaining a

meditation and mindfulness practice may pose challenges. Therefore, we will provide valuable insights and strategies to help you overcome restlessness, wandering thoughts, and other obstacles that may arise during your practice. You will also learn how to sustain motivation and consistency, while seeking support and resources to ensure long-term success.

For those seeking even deeper levels of sleep and profound relaxation, we will explore advanced practices such as yoga nidra, mantra meditation, and the fascinating world of lucid dreaming. Additionally, we will examine the intricate relationship between nutrition, exercise, and sleep, uncovering the mind-body connection and how mindful eating, exercise, and stress reduction techniques can positively impact your sleep quality.

Recognizing that different populations have unique needs, we will dedicate a section to enhancing sleep and relaxation for specific groups. We will discuss meditative practices suitable for children and adolescents, explore the benefits of meditation and mindfulness for older adults, and address the application of these practices in managing sleep disorders.

As we conclude this book, we will recap the key concepts and techniques covered, empowering you to embark on your own meditation and mindfulness journey towards better sleep and relaxation. We will offer encouragement, reminding you of the transformative power that lies within your reach. By embracing these practices, you can transcend the demands of the modern world, finding solace and tranquility within yourself.

Now, let us embark together on this remarkable exploration of meditation and mindfulness practices, as we unlock the gateways to better sleep, profound relaxation, and a more balanced life.

Chapter II: Understanding Sleep and Relaxation

Introduction:

In order to fully grasp the profound impact of meditation and mindfulness on sleep and relaxation, it is essential to understand the science behind sleep, the detrimental effects of stress and anxiety, and the intricate connection between relaxation and overall well-being. In this chapter, we will explore these aspects in depth, shedding light on the importance of achieving quality sleep and cultivating a state of deep relaxation.

I. Exploring the Science of Sleep and its Benefits

A. The Sleep Cycle: Understanding the Stages of Sleep

1. The role of the sleep cycle in promoting restorative sleep

2. Exploring the different stages of sleep: NREM and REM sleep

3. The physiological changes and brain activity during each stage

B. The Importance of Sleep for Physical and Mental Health

1. Restoring the body's energy and repairing cellular damage

2. Enhancing cognitive function, memory consolidation, and learning

3. Regulating mood, emotions, and overall mental well-being

C. The Benefits of Quality Sleep

1. Improved concentration, focus, and productivity

2. Enhanced immune system functioning

3. Lowered risk of chronic conditions, such as heart disease and obesity

II. The Impact of Stress and Anxiety on Sleep Quality

A. Understanding the Stress Response

1. How the body reacts to stress: the fight-or-flight response

2. The role of stress hormones, such as

cortisol, in sleep disruption

3. The cumulative effect of chronic stress on sleep quality

B. Anxiety and Sleep Disturbances

1. The relationship between anxiety disorders and insomnia

2. Racing thoughts and sleep-onset difficulties

3. Interrupted sleep and the impact on overall sleep quality

C. Breaking the Cycle: Addressing Stress and

Anxiety for Better Sleep

1. Stress reduction techniques to promote relaxation before bed

2. Cognitive-behavioral strategies for managing anxiety-related sleep disturbances

3. The role of meditation and mindfulness in alleviating stress and anxiety

III. Uncovering the Connection between Relaxation and Overall Well-being

A. The Physiology of
Relaxation

1. The autonomic
nervous system and its
role in relaxation

2. The relaxation
response: activating
the body's natural
healing mechanisms

3. Lowering heart
rate, blood pressure,
and cortisol levels
through relaxation

B. Psychological
Benefits of Relaxation

1. Reducing
symptoms of anxiety,
depression, and mood
disorders

2. Promoting
emotional resilience

and coping
mechanisms

   3. Enhancing self-
awareness, self-
compassion, and
overall well-being

C. Holistic Wellness:
The Interplay between
Sleep, Relaxation, and
Health

   1. The reciprocal
relationship between
sleep and relaxation

   2. The impact of
sleep and relaxation on
physical, mental, and
emotional health

   3. Creating a
balanced lifestyle that
prioritizes both sleep
and relaxation

Conclusion:

Understanding the
scientific foundations
of sleep, the influence
of stress and anxiety,
and the connection
between relaxation
and overall well-being
lays a strong
foundation for our
exploration of
meditation and
mindfulness practices.
By comprehending the
intricate mechanisms
at play, we can
approach our sleep
and relaxation journey
with greater awareness
and appreciation. In
the subsequent

chapters, we will delve into the fundamental principles of meditation and mindfulness and discover how they can be harnessed to enhance our sleep quality and cultivate profound relaxation.

Chapter III: The
Fundamentals of
Meditation and
Mindfulness

Introduction:

Before diving into the
specific techniques and
practices that can
enhance sleep and
relaxation, it is
important to establish
a solid understanding
of the fundamentals of
meditation and
mindfulness. In this
chapter, we will define
these practices,
explore their historical
and cultural contexts,
and discover how
meditation and

mindfulness contribute to better sleep and relaxation.

      I.   Defining Meditation and Mindfulness

A. Meditation: Cultivating Inner Stillness and Awareness

1. Exploring the essence of meditation as a practice of attention and awareness

2. Differentiating between focused attention and open awareness meditation

3. The role of intention, presence, and non-judgment in meditation

B. Mindfulness: Embracing the Present Moment

1. Defining mindfulness as a state of non-judgmental awareness

2. Cultivating mindfulness through sensory perception and anchoring techniques

3. The connection between mindfulness and self-compassion

C. The Intersection of Meditation and Mindfulness

   1. Recognizing the overlap and synergy between meditation and mindfulness

   2. How meditation cultivates the mindfulness state of being fully present

   3. Embracing both practices for optimal benefits in sleep and relaxation

II.   Brief History and Cultural Context of Meditation and Mindfulness

A. Origins of Meditation: Ancient Roots and Traditions

1. Exploring the historical origins of meditation in ancient civilizations

2. Overview of meditation practices in Eastern traditions (e.g., Buddhism, Hinduism)

3. Influence of Western contemplative practices and secular adaptations

B. Historical Context of Mindfulness

1. The emergence of mindfulness in

Buddhist teachings and philosophy

2. Transmission of mindfulness practices to the West and its integration into healthcare

3. The modern mindfulness movement and its impact on sleep and relaxation

C. Cultural Variations in Meditation and Mindfulness

1. Examining cultural variations in meditation practices worldwide

2. Traditional rituals and approaches to

meditation in different cultures

   3. Appreciating the diverse perspectives and applications of meditation and mindfulness

III.   How Meditation and Mindfulness Contribute to Better Sleep and Relaxation

A. Calming the Mind and Easing Anxiety

   1. Reducing the mental chatter and racing thoughts that disrupt sleep

2. Quieting the mind and alleviating anxiety that can hinder relaxation

3. Building resilience and emotional regulation for improved sleep quality

B. Cultivating Present-Moment Awareness and Relaxation

1. Enhancing the ability to focus on the present moment for better sleep

2. Developing a heightened sense of bodily awareness and relaxation

3. Harnessing mindfulness to

cultivate a state of
calm and tranquility

C. Training the Brain
for Restful Sleep and
Relaxation

   1. Neuroplasticity
and how meditation
reshapes the brain for
improved sleep

   2. Promoting the
production of sleep-
inducing hormones
and neurotransmitters

   3. Establishing a
healthy sleep-wake
cycle through
consistent meditation
practice

Conclusion:

Understanding the fundamentals of meditation and mindfulness is crucial for establishing a solid foundation in our journey towards better sleep and profound relaxation. By defining these practices, exploring their historical and cultural contexts, and recognizing their contributions to sleep and relaxation, we can fully appreciate their transformative power. In the subsequent chapters, we will delve into practical techniques and applications of

meditation and
mindfulness, equipping
ourselves with the
tools to enhance our
sleep quality and
cultivate a state of
deep relaxation.

Chapter IV: Preparing for Better Sleep and Relaxation

Introduction:

Creating the right environment and establishing a consistent routine are essential steps in optimizing sleep and relaxation. In this chapter, we will explore the key factors that contribute to a conducive sleep environment, the importance of a consistent bedtime routine, and how to address common obstacles that may

hinder quality sleep
and relaxation.

I. Creating a
    Conducive
    Sleep
    Environment

A. Setting the Stage for
Restful Sleep

1. Designing a calm
and comfortable
bedroom environment

2. Optimizing lighting,
temperature, and
noise levels for better
sleep

3. Selecting
appropriate bedding,
pillows, and sleep-
supportive accessories

B. Eliminating Sleep Disruptors

   1. Minimizing exposure to electronic devices and blue light before bed

   2. Reducing external stimuli that may disturb sleep (e.g., bright clocks, pets)

   3. Ensuring proper ventilation and air quality for a refreshing sleep environment

C. Incorporating Relaxation Enhancers

   1. Exploring soothing scents, such as lavender or

chamomile, for relaxation

2. Utilizing white noise machines or calming music to promote sleep

3. Incorporating relaxation-promoting elements, such as plants or soft colors

II.   Establishing a Consistent Bedtime Routine

A. The Power of Rituals and Consistency

1. Understanding the importance of a regular sleep schedule

2. Creating a pre-bedtime routine to signal the body and mind for sleep

3. Establishing consistent wake-up times for optimal sleep-wake cycles

B. Wind-Down Activities for Relaxation

1. Engaging in calming activities to promote relaxation before bed

2. Incorporating mindfulness practices into the bedtime routine

3. Avoiding stimulating activities,

caffeine, and heavy meals close to bedtime

C. Promoting Mindful Transition to Sleep

1. Practicing relaxation techniques, such as deep breathing or gentle stretching

2. Incorporating meditation and guided imagery into the bedtime routine

3. Cultivating a sense of gratitude and calmness before transitioning to sleep

III. Addressing Common Obstacles to

Quality Sleep and Relaxation

A. Managing Stress and Anxiety

1. Implementing stress reduction techniques during the day and before bed

2. Journaling or engaging in therapeutic activities to process thoughts and emotions

3. Incorporating mindfulness-based stress reduction practices to alleviate anxiety

B. Dealing with Racing
Thoughts and
Wandering Mind

1. Using relaxation
techniques and
meditation to quiet the
mind

2. Employing
cognitive strategies to
manage intrusive
thoughts

3. Practicing self-
compassion and non-
judgment when the
mind wanders

C. Overcoming Physical
Discomfort

1. Addressing
physical discomfort
through proper sleep
posture and alignment

2. Seeking medical advice for chronic pain or sleep-related issues

3. Exploring relaxation techniques specific to physical relaxation and tension release

Conclusion:

Preparing for better sleep and relaxation involves creating an environment that supports restfulness, establishing a consistent bedtime routine, and addressing common obstacles that may interfere with quality sleep. By optimizing our sleep environment, engaging in a soothing bedtime routine, and finding strategies to overcome sleep disruptors, we can set the stage for improved sleep and deep relaxation. In the subsequent chapters, we will delve into specific techniques and meditation practices that further enhance our ability to achieve restful sleep and profound relaxation.

Chapter V: Techniques for Mindful Sleep

Introduction:

In our quest for better sleep and profound relaxation, incorporating specific mindfulness techniques can greatly enhance our ability to unwind and prepare for a restful night. In this chapter, we will explore three powerful techniques: mindfulness of the breath and body, progressive muscle relaxation, and guided imagery and visualization. These practices can help calm the mind, release tension, and create a peaceful state conducive to deep sleep.

I.   Mindfulness of the Breath and Body

A. Cultivating Breath Awareness

1. The importance of mindful breathing in promoting relaxation

2. Techniques for observing the breath and cultivating present-moment awareness

3. Connecting with the body's natural rhythm to induce relaxation

B. Body Scan Meditation

1. Bringing attention and awareness to different parts of the body

2. Scanning the body systematically to release tension and promote relaxation

3. Cultivating a sense of connection and gratitude for the body's support

C. Mindful Movement for Sleep Preparation

1. Gentle stretching and movement practices to release physical tension

2. Incorporating mindful movement into the bedtime routine

3. Integrating body awareness and relaxation into everyday activities

II.   Progressive Muscle Relaxation for Deep Rest

A. Understanding Progressive Muscle Relaxation (PMR)

1. Exploring the principles and benefits of PMR

2. The connection between muscle tension and sleep disturbances

3. Techniques for consciously releasing muscle tension through PMR

B. Step-by-Step Practice of Progressive Muscle Relaxation

1. Progressive muscle relaxation techniques for the major muscle groups

2. Systematically tensing and relaxing

muscles to induce
deep relaxation

3. Incorporating PMR
into the bedtime
routine for improved
sleep quality

C. Adapting
Progressive Muscle
Relaxation to
Individual Needs

1. Modifying PMR for
specific areas of
tension or discomfort

2. Using guided audio
recordings or
visualization
techniques during PMR

3. Applying PMR
techniques throughout
the day to manage
stress and anxiety

III. Guided Imagery and Visualization for Peaceful Sleep

A. The Power of the Mind-Body Connection

1. Understanding the influence of visualization on the relaxation response

2. The role of guided imagery in redirecting thoughts and calming the mind

3. Harnessing the imagination to create a peaceful sleep environment

B. Creating a Guided Imagery Script for Sleep

1. Crafting a soothing narrative for relaxation and sleep

2. Incorporating sensory details to enhance the visualization experience

3. Using imagery to create a mental sanctuary for restful sleep

C. Utilizing Guided Imagery and Visualization Resources

1. Exploring guided meditation apps,

recordings, or online resources

2. Customizing guided imagery scripts to suit personal preferences

3. Integrating guided visualization into the bedtime routine for enhanced relaxation

Conclusion:

Techniques for mindful sleep, such as mindfulness of the breath and body, progressive muscle relaxation, and guided imagery and visualization, provide powerful tools for calming the mind, releasing physical tension, and creating a peaceful state conducive to deep sleep. By incorporating these practices into our bedtime routine, we can cultivate a sense of tranquility and prepare our minds and bodies for restful sleep. In the subsequent chapters, we will continue to explore meditation practices specifically tailored for relaxation, further deepening our journey toward better sleep and profound relaxation.

Chapter VI: Meditation Practices for Relaxation

Introduction:

Meditation is a powerful tool for cultivating relaxation, promoting self-awareness, and fostering a deep sense of calm. In this chapter, we will explore three meditation practices specifically designed to enhance relaxation: mindful awareness of thoughts and emotions, loving-kindness meditation for self-compassion and stress reduction, and body scan meditation for releasing tension and promoting relaxation. These practices will allow you to deepen your connection with yourself, cultivate compassion, and create a state of profound relaxation.

I.   Mindful Awareness of Thoughts and Emotions

A. Understanding the Role of Mindfulness in Relaxation

1. The relationship between mindfulness and calming the mind

2. Cultivating non-judgmental awareness of thoughts and emotions

3. Embracing mindfulness as a tool for relaxation and stress reduction

B. Developing Mindful Awareness of Thoughts

1. Observing thoughts as passing mental events without attachment

2. Practicing non-reactivity and letting go of ruminative thinking

3. Cultivating a spacious and calm

mental state through
mindfulness

C. Embracing Emotions
with Mindful Presence

1. Recognizing and
accepting emotions
without judgment

2. Allowing emotions
to arise and pass with
mindful awareness

3. Using mindfulness
to regulate emotional
responses and
promote relaxation

II.   Loving-
        Kindness
        Meditation for
        Self-
        Compassion

and Stress
Reduction

A. The Power of Loving-Kindness Meditation

1. Understanding the principles and benefits of loving-kindness meditation

2. Cultivating a sense of kindness, compassion, and well-wishing

3. Harnessing the practice to reduce stress and enhance relaxation

B. Extending Loving-Kindness to Oneself

1. Generating
feelings of self-
compassion and self-
acceptance

2. Offering loving-
kindness phrases or
affirmations to oneself

3. Using loving-
kindness meditation as
a tool for self-soothing
and relaxation

C. Expanding Loving-
Kindness to Others

1. Cultivating a sense
of connectedness and
empathy towards
others

2. Offering loving-
kindness and well-
wishes to loved ones
and acquaintances

3. Promoting a state
of relaxation and
harmony through
loving-kindness
practice

III.   Body Scan
Meditation for
Releasing
Tension and
Promoting
Relaxation

A. The Benefits of Body
Scan Meditation

1. Understanding the
mind-body connection
in relaxation

2. Cultivating body
awareness to release
tension and promote
relaxation

3. Deepening the connection between mind, body, and relaxation

B. Practicing a Guided Body Scan Meditation

1. Systematically scanning the body from head to toe with awareness

2. Observing physical sensations and releasing tension with each scan

3. Allowing the body to relax fully and promoting a state of deep relaxation

C. Incorporating Body Scan Meditation into Daily Life

  1. Mini body scan meditations for quick relaxation breaks throughout the day

  2. Using body scan techniques to release tension in specific areas of the body

  3. Integrating body scan meditation into the bedtime routine for restful sleep

Conclusion:

Meditation practices specifically focused on relaxation, such as mindful awareness of

thoughts and
emotions, loving-
kindness meditation
for self-compassion
and stress reduction,
and body scan
meditation for
releasing tension,
provide powerful tools
for cultivating
profound relaxation
and inner peace. By
incorporating these
practices into your
daily routine, you can
deepen your self-
awareness, foster
compassion, and
experience a state of
deep relaxation. In the
subsequent chapters,
we will continue to
explore meditation and
mindfulness

techniques to further
enhance your sleep
and relaxation journey.

Chapter VII: Integrating Meditation and Mindfulness into Daily Life

Introduction:

The benefits of meditation and mindfulness extend far beyond dedicated practice sessions. By integrating these practices into our daily lives, we can enhance our overall well-being, manage stress and anxiety, and cultivate a deeper sense of relaxation. In this chapter, we will explore three key aspects of integrating meditation and mindfulness into daily life: applying mindfulness to daily activities for increased relaxation, cultivating gratitude and joy through mindfulness, and managing stress and anxiety through regular meditation practice.

I. Applying Mindfulness to Daily Activities for Increased Relaxation

A. The Power of Present-Moment Awareness

1. Bringing mindful awareness to everyday activities for relaxation

2. Cultivating a sense of mindfulness during routine tasks

3. Transforming mundane activities into opportunities for relaxation and presence

B. Mindful Eating for Nourishment and Relaxation

1. Engaging in mindful eating to enhance digestion and relaxation

2. Savoring each bite and tuning into the

body's hunger and
fullness cues

   3. Cultivating
gratitude and
appreciation for the
nourishment received

C. Mindful Movement
for Relaxation and
Stress Reduction

   1. Incorporating
mindfulness into
physical activities like
walking or yoga

   2. Noticing
sensations, breath, and
body movements
during exercise

   3. Using mindful
movement as a means
to release tension and
promote relaxation

II.   Cultivating Gratitude and Joy through Mindfulness

A. Gratitude as a Path to Relaxation

1. Understanding the link between gratitude and overall well-being

2. Cultivating gratitude through mindful reflection and appreciation

3. Using gratitude practices to shift focus towards positivity and relaxation

B. Joyful Moments of Mindfulness

1. Noticing and savoring moments of joy and happiness in daily life

2. Cultivating mindfulness of positive experiences to enhance relaxation

3. Letting go of expectations and embracing the present moment with joy

C. Loving-Kindness Meditation for Connection and Relaxation

1. Extending loving-kindness and well-

wishes to oneself and others

2. Cultivating a sense of interconnectedness and compassion through meditation

3. Promoting relaxation and a deeper sense of peace through loving-kindness

III. Managing Stress and Anxiety through Regular Meditation Practice

A. The Role of
Meditation in Stress
Reduction

   1. Understanding the
impact of stress on
sleep and relaxation

   2. Using meditation
as a tool to manage
stress and anxiety

   3. Cultivating a sense
of calm and relaxation
through regular
practice

B. Mindfulness-Based
Stress Reduction
Techniques

   1. Incorporating
mindfulness into stress
management
strategies

2. Breathing techniques and body awareness to reduce stress responses

3. Mindful coping mechanisms for navigating challenging situations

C. Establishing a Sustainable Meditation Routine

1. Setting realistic goals for regular meditation practice

2. Overcoming obstacles and maintaining consistency

3. Utilizing meditation resources

and seeking support
for long-term success

Conclusion:

Integrating meditation
and mindfulness into
our daily lives offers a
powerful means to
increase relaxation,
cultivate gratitude and
joy, and manage stress
and anxiety. By
applying mindfulness
to daily activities,
embracing gratitude
and joyful moments,
and establishing a
regular meditation
practice, we can
enhance our overall
well-being and
experience a greater

sense of calm and relaxation throughout our lives. In the subsequent chapters, we will explore advanced practices and further techniques to deepen our sleep and relaxation journey.

Chapter VIII:
Overcoming Challenges and Sustaining Practice

Introduction:

Embarking on a meditation and mindfulness journey for better sleep and relaxation is a transformative endeavor. However, it is not without its challenges. In this chapter, we will explore three key aspects of overcoming challenges and sustaining your practice: dealing with restlessness and wandering thoughts during meditation, strategies for maintaining motivation and consistency, and seeking support and resources for long-term success. By addressing these challenges head-on, you can navigate the obstacles and cultivate a sustainable practice that enhances your sleep and relaxation.

I. Dealing with Restlessness and Wandering Thoughts during Meditation

A. Understanding the Nature of Restlessness and Wandering Thoughts

1. Recognizing restlessness as a common experience during meditation

2. Acknowledging the nature of the wandering mind and its impact on relaxation

3. Cultivating acceptance and non-judgment in the face of restlessness and thoughts

B. Techniques for Managing Restlessness and Wandering Thoughts

1. Anchoring techniques to redirect attention and calm the mind

2. Noticing and labeling thoughts without attachment or judgment

3. Embracing the impermanent nature of thoughts and returning to the present moment

C. Cultivating Patience and Persistence in Meditation

1. Understanding that restlessness and wandering thoughts are part of the process

2. Developing patience and self-

compassion during
meditation practice

3. Trusting in the
transformative power
of consistent effort
over time

II.   Strategies for
Maintaining
Motivation
and
Consistency

A. Setting Realistic
Goals and Expectations

1. Defining
achievable goals for
your meditation and
mindfulness practice

2. Cultivating a
balanced perspective

on progress and
growth

   3. Celebrating small
milestones and
recognizing the
benefits of regular
practice

B. Establishing a
Personalized Routine

   1. Identifying the
best time and duration
for your meditation
practice

   2. Creating a
dedicated space for
meditation to enhance
consistency

   3. Integrating
meditation into your
daily routine for long-
term sustainability

C. Exploring Variety in Your Practice

1. Incorporating different meditation techniques to keep your practice fresh

2. Exploring guided meditations, visualization, or mantra-based practices

3. Adapting your practice to suit your evolving needs and interests

III.   Seeking Support and Resources for Long-Term Success

A. Engaging in
Community and Group
Practices

1. Joining meditation
groups or communities
for support and
connection

2. Participating in
group meditation
sessions or retreats for
inspiration

3. Sharing
experiences and
insights with like-
minded individuals

B. Utilizing Technology
and Meditation Apps

1. Exploring
meditation apps and

online resources for guidance and support

2. Incorporating technology into your practice with guided meditations or timers

3. Tracking progress and staying accountable with meditation apps

C. Seeking Guidance from Teachers or Mentors

1. Finding a meditation teacher or mentor to deepen your practice

2. Seeking guidance and clarification on challenges or questions that arise

3. Embracing the wisdom and guidance of experienced practitioners

Conclusion:

Overcoming challenges and sustaining your meditation and mindfulness practice is crucial for long-term success in enhancing sleep and relaxation. By adopting strategies to manage restlessness and wandering thoughts, maintaining motivation and consistency, and seeking support and resources, you can navigate obstacles and cultivate a sustainable practice. Remember that this journey is a process, and with patience, persistence, and the right tools, you can continue to deepen your practice and reap the benefits of improved sleep and profound relaxation. In the subsequent chapters, we will explore advanced practices and techniques to further enhance your sleep and relaxation journey.

Chapter IX: Advanced
Practices for Deep
Sleep and Profound
Relaxation

Introduction:

As you continue your
journey toward better
sleep and profound
relaxation, it's time to
explore advanced
practices that can
further enhance your
experience. In this
chapter, we will delve
into three powerful
techniques: yoga nidra
for conscious sleep and
rejuvenation, mantra
meditation for
transcending mental
chatter, and exploring

lucid dreaming for enhanced sleep experiences. These practices offer unique pathways to deep relaxation, expanded awareness, and transformative sleep.

I. Yoga Nidra for Conscious Sleep and Rejuvenation

A. Understanding Yoga Nidra

1. Exploring the concept and benefits of yoga nidra

2. The connection between conscious

sleep and deep relaxation

  3. How yoga nidra can contribute to improved sleep and overall well-being

B. Practicing Yoga Nidra for Deep Relaxation

  1. Preparing for a yoga nidra session with a relaxed body and mind

  2. Guided awareness of body sensations and breath during the practice

  3. Cultivating a state of conscious relaxation and rejuvenation

C. Integrating Yoga Nidra into Your Sleep Routine

   1. Incorporating yoga nidra into your bedtime routine for restful sleep

   2. Using recorded yoga nidra sessions or practicing with a guide

   3. Adapting yoga nidra techniques to suit your unique needs and preferences

II.   Mantra Meditation for Transcending Mental Chatter

A. Understanding Mantra Meditation

   1. Exploring the purpose and benefits of mantra meditation

   2. The role of repetitive sounds or phrases in calming the mind

   3. Using mantras to transcend mental chatter and enter a state of deep relaxation

B. Practicing Mantra Meditation for Sleep Enhancement

   1. Choosing a mantra that resonates with your intention for better sleep

2. Repetition and focus on the mantra to quiet the mind and induce relaxation

3. Allowing the vibration of the mantra to guide you into a restful state of sleep

C. Incorporating Mantra Meditation into Daily Life

1. Using mantra meditation during waking hours to reduce stress and anxiety

2. Connecting with the soothing power of mantras during challenging moments

3. Infusing daily activities with

mindfulness and
mantra recitation for
relaxation

III.   Exploring Lucid
        Dreaming for
        Enhanced
        Sleep
        Experiences

A. Understanding Lucid
Dreaming

   1. Exploring the
concept and potential
benefits of lucid
dreaming

   2. Becoming aware
within the dream state
for conscious
exploration

   3. How lucid
dreaming can

contribute to deeper sleep and transformative experiences

B. Techniques for Inducing Lucid Dreams

1. Practicing reality checks and maintaining dream journals for increased dream awareness

2. Using mnemonic induction techniques (MILD) to enhance lucid dreaming

3. Incorporating visualization and intention-setting before sleep for lucidity

C. Harnessing Lucid
Dreams for Relaxation
and Self-Exploration

1. Cultivating
relaxation and serenity
within lucid dreams

2. Engaging in
creative visualization
and problem-solving
during lucid dreaming

3. Using lucid dreams
as a platform for
personal growth and
spiritual exploration

Conclusion:

Advanced practices
such as yoga nidra,
mantra meditation,
and lucid dreaming
offer profound

opportunities for deep sleep and transformative relaxation. By incorporating these techniques into your sleep routine and daily life, you can experience heightened awareness, transcendental experiences, and enhanced relaxation. As you continue your journey, embrace these advanced practices and explore their potential for creating a truly restful and transformative sleep experience. In the subsequent chapters, we will further explore the

mind-body connection
and techniques to
optimize sleep and
relaxation.

Chapter X: The Mind-Body Connection: Nutrition, Exercise, and Sleep

Introduction:

The mind and body are intricately connected, and the choices we make regarding our nutrition, exercise, and stress management can significantly impact our sleep and relaxation. In this chapter, we will explore the mind-body connection and its influence on sleep quality. Specifically, we will focus on three key areas: how diet and nutrition influence sleep quality, the impact of exercise on sleep and relaxation, and mindfulness-based stress reduction techniques for better sleep.

I. How Diet and Nutrition Influence Sleep Quality

A. Understanding the Relationship Between Diet and Sleep

1. Exploring the connection between certain foods and sleep quality

2. The role of macronutrients and micronutrients in promoting relaxation

3. The impact of caffeine, alcohol, and late-night eating on sleep patterns

B. Promoting Sleep-Friendly Foods and Beverages

1. Foods rich in tryptophan, magnesium, and calcium for relaxation

2. Herbal teas and natural sleep aids that support restful sleep

3. Incorporating a balanced and nutritious diet for overall sleep health

C. Establishing Healthy Eating Habits for Better Sleep

   1. Timing meals and snacks to optimize digestion and sleep cycles

   2. Mindful eating practices to reduce stress and promote relaxation

   3. Maintaining a consistent meal routine to support a healthy sleep-wake cycle

II.   Exercise and Its Impact on Sleep and Relaxation

A. The Relationship Between Exercise and Sleep

1. Exploring the benefits of regular exercise on sleep quality

2. Understanding the role of physical activity in reducing stress and anxiety

3. The impact of exercise timing on sleep patterns and energy levels

B. Choosing the Right Exercise for Sleep Enhancement

1. Aerobic exercises that promote

relaxation and improve sleep quality

2. Mind-body practices such as yoga or tai chi for stress reduction

3. Finding a balance between physical activity and relaxation for optimal sleep

C. Creating an Exercise Routine that Supports Sleep

1. Establishing a consistent exercise schedule for better sleep regulation

2. Avoiding vigorous exercise close to bedtime to promote relaxation

3. Incorporating relaxation techniques post-exercise to facilitate restful sleep

III.   Mindfulness-Based Stress Reduction Techniques for Better Sleep

A. Understanding the Impact of Stress on Sleep

1. Exploring the relationship between stress and sleep disturbances

2. The role of chronic stress in disrupting sleep patterns

3. Recognizing the
importance of stress
reduction for better
sleep and relaxation

B. Mindfulness-Based
Stress Reduction
(MBSR) Techniques

1. Practicing
mindfulness
meditation for stress
reduction and
relaxation

2. Incorporating
mindful breathing and
body scans to calm the
nervous system

3. Cultivating self-
compassion and
acceptance as tools for
stress reduction

C. Integrating Mindfulness-Based Stress Reduction into Daily Life

1. Creating a daily mindfulness practice for stress management

2. Applying mindfulness techniques during stressful situations for relaxation

3. Using mindfulness as a tool to promote a peaceful mind and better sleep

Conclusion:

The mind-body connection plays a vital role in our sleep and relaxation. By understanding how diet and nutrition influence sleep quality, incorporating regular exercise for better sleep, and utilizing mindfulness-based stress reduction techniques, we can optimize our sleep and relaxation journey. Through conscious choices and practices, we can create a harmonious mind-body balance that promotes restful sleep and profound relaxation. In the subsequent chapters, we will continue to explore techniques and practices to further

enhance your sleep
and relaxation
experience.

Chapter XI: Enhancing
Sleep and Relaxation
for Specific Populations

Introduction:

The benefits of
meditation and
mindfulness practices
extend to individuals of
all ages and
backgrounds. In this
chapter, we will
explore how to
enhance sleep and
relaxation for specific
populations. We will
focus on three key
areas: meditative
practices for children
and adolescents,
meditation and
mindfulness for older

adults, and addressing sleep disorders through meditation and mindfulness. By tailoring these practices to the unique needs of these populations, we can cultivate a deeper sense of well-being and improve sleep quality.

I.   Meditative Practices for Children and Adolescents

A. Introducing Mindfulness to Children and Adolescents

1. The benefits of mindfulness for children's and adolescents' sleep and relaxation

2. Making mindfulness accessible and engaging for younger age groups

3. Incorporating age-appropriate meditation techniques and activities

B. Mindful Breathing and Body Awareness for Children

1. Teaching children to connect with their breath as a relaxation tool

2. Cultivating body
awareness through
simple movements and
guided imagery

3. Incorporating
mindfulness into daily
routines and activities
for children

C. Mindfulness-Based
Practices for
Adolescents

1. Addressing stress
and sleep disturbances
in adolescents through
mindfulness

2. Guided meditation
and mindful self-
compassion for
emotional well-being

3. Empowering
adolescents with

mindfulness tools for better sleep and relaxation

II. Meditation and Mindfulness for Older Adults

A. Recognizing the Unique Needs of Older Adults for Sleep and Relaxation

1. Understanding age-related sleep changes and challenges

2. The role of mindfulness in managing sleep disturbances in older adults

3. Adapting
meditation practices to
suit the physical and
cognitive abilities of
older adults

B. Gentle Movement
and Mindfulness for
Older Adults

1. Incorporating
gentle yoga or seated
meditation for
relaxation

2. Mindful walking or
slow movements for
promoting relaxation
and sleep

3. Enhancing body
awareness and self-
care practices for
better sleep hygiene

C. Cultivating
Mindfulness for Aging
Well

   1. Embracing
mindfulness as a tool
for accepting and
adapting to changes

   2. Mindfulness
practices for managing
age-related stress and
anxiety

   3. Utilizing
mindfulness
techniques to enhance
sleep quality and
overall well-being

   III.   Addressing
           Sleep
           Disorders
           through
           Meditation

and
Mindfulness

A. Understanding the Link Between Sleep Disorders and Mental Well-being

1. Exploring the relationship between sleep disorders and stress/anxiety

2. The role of meditation and mindfulness in managing sleep disorders

3. Addressing the root causes of sleep disorders through holistic approaches

B. Mindfulness-Based Cognitive Therapy for Insomnia (MBCT-I)

1. Utilizing mindfulness to shift patterns of rumination and worry

2. Mindfulness techniques for managing racing thoughts and bedtime anxiety

3. Cultivating a peaceful and calm state of mind for improved sleep quality

C. Meditation Practices for Sleep Apnea and Restless Legs Syndrome

1. Exploring specific meditation techniques for sleep apnea and relaxation

2. Addressing restless legs syndrome through mindfulness and gentle movements

3. Developing a personalized meditation routine to manage sleep disorders

Conclusion:

Enhancing sleep and relaxation for specific populations requires tailoring meditation and mindfulness practices to their unique needs. By introducing mindfulness to children and adolescents, incorporating meditation and mindfulness for older adults, and addressing sleep disorders through targeted techniques, we can promote better sleep and relaxation for these groups. By embracing the diverse needs of different populations, we foster a more inclusive and effective approach to sleep and relaxation. In the subsequent chapters, we will continue to explore

techniques and
practices to further
enhance your sleep
and relaxation
experience.

Chapter XII: Conclusion

Introduction:

Congratulations on completing this journey into the world of meditation and mindfulness practices for better sleep and relaxation. Throughout this book, we have explored various techniques, concepts, and strategies to enhance your sleep and promote deep relaxation. In this concluding chapter, we will recap the key concepts and techniques covered, provide encouragement for readers to embark on their own meditation and mindfulness journey, and reflect on the transformative power of sleep and relaxation through meditation.

I.   Recap of Key Concepts and Techniques Covered in the Book

In this book, we have delved into a wide range of topics related to meditation, mindfulness, sleep, and relaxation. Let's take a moment to

recap the key concepts
and techniques
covered:

1. Understanding the
importance of sleep
and relaxation in
today's fast-paced
world

2. Exploring the science
of sleep and its
benefits

3. Uncovering the
impact of stress and
anxiety on sleep
quality

4. Defining meditation
and mindfulness and
their contributions to
better sleep and
relaxation

5. Creating a conducive sleep environment and establishing a consistent bedtime routine

6. Techniques for mindful sleep, including mindfulness of the breath and body, progressive muscle relaxation, and guided imagery

7. Meditation practices for relaxation, such as mindful awareness of thoughts and emotions, loving-kindness meditation, and body scan meditation

8. Integrating meditation and mindfulness into daily

life through mindful activities, gratitude practices, and stress reduction techniques

9. Overcoming challenges and sustaining your meditation practice through managing restlessness, maintaining motivation, and seeking support

10. Exploring advanced practices for deep sleep and profound relaxation, including yoga nidra, mantra meditation, and lucid dreaming

11. Understanding the mind-body connection and its influence on

sleep, including the impact of diet, exercise, and stress reduction techniques

12. Enhancing sleep and relaxation for specific populations, such as children and adolescents, older adults, and individuals with sleep disorders

II. Encouragement for Readers to Embark on Their Own Meditation and Mindfulness Journey

As you reach the end
of this book, we want
to encourage you to
embark on your own
meditation and
mindfulness journey.
Remember that the
path to better sleep
and profound
relaxation is unique for
each individual.
Embrace the
techniques and
practices that resonate
with you, and feel free
to experiment and
adapt them to suit
your needs and
preferences. Stay
patient and
compassionate with
yourself as you
navigate the challenges
and joys that come

with establishing a regular practice. The transformative power of meditation and mindfulness awaits you as you cultivate a deeper connection with yourself and the present moment.

III.   Final Thoughts on the Transformative Power of Sleep and Relaxation through Meditation

Sleep and relaxation are not merely a means to an end but an essential part of our well-being. By incorporating meditation and mindfulness practices into your life, you have the opportunity to unlock the transformative power of sleep and relaxation. As you learn to quiet the mind, release tension, and cultivate present-moment awareness, you pave the way for deeper sleep, improved mental and physical health, and a greater sense of overall well-being. Remember that the benefits of this journey extend beyond the moments of practice and into your daily life. Embrace the wisdom and insights gained through this exploration, and carry them with you as you continue your path toward better sleep, profound relaxation, and a more mindful way of living.

Conclusion:

Thank you for joining us on this journey of meditation and mindfulness practices for better sleep and relaxation. We hope that this book has provided you with valuable insights, techniques, and

inspiration to enhance
your sleep and
relaxation experience.
Remember to be
patient, kind, and
consistent in your
practice. Embrace the
transformative power
of meditation and
mindfulness as you
navigate the challenges
and joys of your own
journey. May you find
deep sleep, profound
relaxation, and an
abundance of peace
and well-being. Sleep
well and live mindfully.